Table of Contents

A flexitarian or semi-vegetarian diet (SVD) is one that is primarily vegetarian with the occasional inclusion of meat or fish. Of late, there appears to be an increasing movement toward this practice. There has not been a recent update on these diets from a health perspective. Using the National Centre for Biotechnology Information PubMed database, a search was made for all studies published between 2000 and 2016 that met defined inclusion criteria. A total of 25 studies were located with 12 focusing on body weight and diet quality. There was emerging evidence suggestive of benefits for body weight, improved markers of metabolic health, blood pressure, and reduced risk of type 2 diabetes. SVD may also have a role to play in the treatment of inflammatory bowel diseases, such as Crohn's disease. Given that there is a higher tendency for females to be flexitarian yet males are more likely to overconsume meat, there is a clear need to communicate the potential health benefits of these diets to males.

BREAKFAST

1. Waffles with Grilled Nectarines

Prep Time: 10 Minutes

Cook Time: 15 Minutes

Servings: 6

Ingredients

For The Cashew Cream:

- 140 g unsalted cashews
- 125 ml dairy-free milk
- 3 tbsp maple syrup
- 1 tbsp lemon juice
- ¼ teaspoon salt

For The Waffles:

- 250 g plain flour
- 1 tbsp sugar
- 4 teaspoons baking powder
- ½ teaspoon salt

- 400 ml dairy-free milk

- 60 ml neutral-tasting vegetable oil

- 1 tablespoon apple cider vinegar

- 1 teaspoon vanilla extract

Toppings:

- 3 nectarines

- Vegetable oil

- Granola

- Mint leaves

Instructions

1. Place cashews in a bowl. Cover with boiling water. Set aside to soak for 20 minutes.

2. Drain the cashews. Place in the bowl of a blender with 125ml [US 1/2 cup] dairy-free milk, maple syrup, lemon juice, and salt. Whizz until smooth. Set aside.

3. To make the waffles, stir together the flour, sugar, baking powder, and salt in a large mixing bowl.

4. In a separate bowl, mix together the dairy-free milk, oil, cider vinegar, and vanilla extract.

5. Whisk the wet ingredients into the dry ingredients until you have a smooth batter without lumps.

6. Pre-heat a greased waffe iron.

7. Spread some of the waffle batter so that to cover 3/4 of the waffle plate. Close and cook for 3 to 5 minutes until crisp and golden. Conveniently, my waffle maker beeps to let me know the waffles are ready!

8. When done transfer the waffle to a rack and keep warm while you are making the rest of the waffles.

9. In the meantime, heat a greased griddle pan on high heat. Cut the nectarines in half and remove the stones. Grill the nectarines face down until softened, and set aside.

10. Serve each waffle topped with a nectarine half, some cashew cream, a sprinkle of your favourite granola, and a few sprigs of mint.

Prep Time: 10 Minutes

Cook Time: 20 Minutes

Servings: 12

Ingredients

- 100 g rolled oats
- 240 ml dairy-free milk
- 1 tablespoon milled chia seeds
- 150 g plain flour
- 1 teaspoon baking powder
- 1 teaspoon bicarbonate of soda
- 150 g light brown soft sugar
- 120 ml vegetable oil
- 1 ½ teaspoon vanilla extract
- 1 overripe mashed banana (around 100g / 1/3 US cup of flesh)
- 150 g frozen cherries,, halved
- 75 g dark chocolate chips

For The Oat Topping:

- 2 tablespoons rolled oats

- 2 tablespoons plain flour
- 2 tablespoons light soft brown sugar
- 1 tablespoon vegetable oil (neutral tasting)

Instructions

1. Mix together the rolled oats, dairy-free milk and milled chia seeds. Set aside for 20 minutes.
2. Prepare the oat topping by mixing together in a small bowl 2 tablespoons rolled oats, 2 tablespoons plain flour, 2 tablespoons light soft brown sugar and 1 tablespoon of vegetable oil. Set aside.
3. After the oats have been soaking for 10 minutes, preheat the oven to Fan 180°C / 200°C/400°F/Gas 6. Place 12 large paper baking cases in a muffin tin.
4. In a medium bowl, mix together the plain flour, baking powder, bicarbonate of soda and light brown soft sugar.
5. In a separate bowl mix together the vegetable oil, vanilla extract and mashed banana.
6. Mix the dry and wet ingredients until well combined. Fold in the cherries and chocolate chips.

7. Spoon the batter evenly into each muffin paper baking case in the muffin tin. Share the oat topping evenly between the muffins

8. Place in the oven for around 25mins. Insert a skewer to check they are cooked. A skewer should come out clean.

Prep Time: 5 Minutes

Cook Time: 20 Minutes

Servings: 2

Ingredients

- olive oil
- 1 red onion
- 4 small portobello mushrooms or 2 large
- 2 to matoes
- 1 garlic clove crushed
- 2 handfuls of spinach
- 390 g firm tofu
- 2 tablespoons nutritional yeast
- 1/2 teaspoon garlic powder
- 1/2 teaspoon salt
- 1 tsp dried thyme
- 1/2 teaspoon turmeric
- 2 Tbsp non-dairy milk

To Serve:

- slices of your favorite bread

- selection of your favourite sauces

Instructions

1. Heat some olive oil in a frying pan. Add finely chopped onion and fry gently until soft. When done, set aside in a bowl.
2. Add some more oil to the frying pan. Cut tomatoes in half and place cut-side down in the pan. Add mushrooms to the pan. Cook all together until tender, flipping the vegetables from time to time.
3. In the meantime prepare the tofu scramble. Drain the tofu. Place in another pan and mash with a fork into a scramble. Add the turmeric, garlic powder, nutritional yeast, dried thyme, salt and non-dairy milk. Mix well. Cook under medium heat, stirring often, until golden. Keep warm under low heat while you finish the rest.
4. Once the tomatoes and mushrooms are cooked, push them to the side of the pan to make space for the spinach. Add reserved onion and garlic to the pan, followed by the spinach. Cook until wilted.
5. Share the tofu scramble evenly between two plates. Add two tomato halves to each plate, alongside some mushrooms and spinach. Serve hot with some slices

of your favourite bread toasted and sauces of your choice.

Prep Time: 25 Minutes

Cook Time: 30 Minutes

Servings: 4

Ingredients

- 1 tofu press
- 1 mixing bowl
- 1 large frying pan
- 400 g extra-firm tofu
- 200 g basmati rice
- 2 tbsp melted coconut oil
- 1 medium onion
- 250 g mushrooms
- 125 g frozen peas

For The Sauce:

- 1 1/2 tbsp Gochujang paste (Sunchang Red Pepper Paste)
- 2 tbsp tamari sauce
- 1 tbsp rice vinegar
- 2 tbsp light brown sugar

- 200 ml light coconut milk
- Lemon juice
- Salt

To Serve:

- Rice
- Spring onion
- Red chilli

Instructions

1. Press the tofu for around 15 minutes to extract as much water as possible. You can use a tofu press or wrap the tofu in a clean towel and press it between 2 plates by securely placing something heavy on top. When done, cut the drained tofu into 1.5-cm / 1/2-inch dice.
2. In the meantime, start cooking the curry.
3. In a mixing bowl, stir together the Gochujang paste, tamari sauce, rice vinegar and brown sugar. Set aside
4. Cut the onion into small dice. Roughly chop the mushrooms.
5. Start cooking the rice.

6. Heat the coconut oil under medium heat in a large frying pan. Add the diced onion and fry until soft, about 5 minutes.

7. Add the mushrooms to the pan and fry for another 5 minutes.

8. Add the tofu and frozen peas. Mix in the Gochujang sauce and coconut milk. Stirring often, cook for a further 5 minutes until the peas are cooked.

9. Season to taste with a splash of lemon juice and some salt if needed.

10. Serve on rice, topped with a sprinkle of sliced spring onions and some chilli.

Prep Time: 25 Minutes

Cook Time: 10 Minutes

Servings: 4

Ingredients

- 2 mixing bowls
- 1 mandoline
- 4 skewer sticks

For The Kebabs:

- 250 g halloumi
- 1 medium yellow courgette
- 1 medium green courgette
- ½ orange pepper
- 4 large cherry tomatoes
- 2 Tbsp olive oil
- 1 tsp dry thyme
- Extra olive oil to drizzle

For The Salsa:

- 400 g watermelon flesh

- 100 g cooked black beans, drained and rinsed
- 3 Tbsp finely chopped mint leaves
- 2 Tbsp finely chopped coriander leaves
- 3 Tbsp finely chopped basil leaves
- ½ red onion
- 1 grated garlic clove
- 2 Tbsp lemon juice
- 2 Tbsp olive oil
- ½ to 1 red chilli (to taste)
- Salt to taste

To Serve:

- 4 flatbreads
- 2 handfuls of rocket leaves

Instructions

1. If you are using wooden skewers, soak them in water beforehand for 20 minutes or more.
2. Cut the halloumi black into 8 equal cubes.
3. Using a mandoline on the smallest setting, cut the courgettes lengthwise into thin slices. If you do not have a mandoline, you can use a vegetable peeler or a

very sharp knife. The slices should be thin enough that they can be bent without breaking.

4. Cut the pepper into 8 equal cubes.

5. Place the halloumi, courgettes, pepper and tomatoes in a mixing bowl. Toss is 2 tablespoons of olive oil and 1 teaspoon of dry thyme. Set aside.

6. To make the salsa, cut the watermelon into 1cm / 0.4-inch dice. Place in a salad bowl with the black beans, chopped herbs, finely diced red onion, and garlic. Toss in 2 tablespoons of olive oil and 2 tablespoons of lemon juice. Season to taste with salt. Add the chopped chilli if using. Set aside.

7. To make the skewers, place 1 pepper cube through one kebab stick, followed by 1 cube of halloumi, some green and yellow courgettes slices folded onto themselves, 1 tomato, some more green and yellow courgettes, another halloumi cube and finish with a pepper cube. Repeat with the other 3 kebabs.

8. Put the grill on high. Drizzle the kebabs with some olive oil and cook for 6-8 minutes, turning them over after 3-4 minutes to make sure they are evenly cooked.

9. Serve these grilled halloumi kebabs with flatbread topped with some watermelon salsa.

Prep Time: 05 Minutes

Cook Time: 15 Minutes

Servings: 2

Ingredients

- 2 saucepans
- baking tray
- gril
- 12 asparagus
- 2 organic eggs
- 90 g feta cheese
- 2 slices of sourdough bread
- olive oil
- small handful of almonds – roughly chopped
- zest of 1 unwaxed lemon
- 1 tsp chopped mint leaves
- 1 tsp chopped parsley
- 1 tsp chopped chives
- Salt & pepper

Instructions

1. Put the grill on.
2. Prepare chopped herbs. Crumble feta cheese.
3. Heat some water in a small saucepan. Add some vinegar in the water. When water is boiling, reduce the heat to a gentle simmer.
4. Place the asparagus on a baking tray with a drizzle of olive oil on top. Roast for 5-8mins depending on size. Keep an eye so they do not burn.
5. To make the poached eggs, crack the first egg and place in a ramekin.
6. Whisk the water to create a gentle whirpool.
7. Delicately place the egg into the simmering water.
8. Poach the first egg for around 2-3 minutes.
9. Remove poached egg with a perforated spoon and drain on kitchen paper.
10. Poach second egg.
11. Toast the bread in the meantime.
12. Place some crumbled feta on each slice of bread. Top each slice with 6 asparagus.
13. Top with poached egg, mixed herbs, sliced almonds, lemon zest and a drizzle of olive oil.
14. Season to taste with salt & pepper.

Prep Time: 20 Minutes

Cook Time: 25 Minutes

Servings: 12

Ingredients

- 2 mixing bowls
- muffin tin
- 1 chia egg [1 Tbsp ground chia seeds + 3 Tbsp of water] / or 1 organic egg
- 125 g plain flour
- 125 g wholemeal spelt flour
- 125 g golden caster sugar
- 1 tsp baking powder
- 1 tsp baking soda
- 1/2 tsp salt
- 1 tsp ground nutmeg
- 2 Tbsp of lemon juice + zest
- 2-3 overripe bananas [250g / 8.8 oz]
- 60 ml vegetable oil
- 125 ml almond milk
- 125 g fresh blueberry

Instructions

1. Preheat the oven to Fan 180°C / 200°C/400°F/Gas 6. Place 12 large paper baking cases in a muffin tin.
2. Prepare chia egg by mixing 1 Tbsp of ground chia seeds with 3 Tbsp of water. Set aside for 10 mins.
3. In a large bowl, mix together flours, sugar, baking powder, baking soda, salt, ground nutmeg and lemon zest.
4. In a separate bowl, mash bananas with a fork. Whisk in lemon juice, chia egg, vegetable oil and almond milk.
5. Add the dry ingredients to the wet ingredients and mix until well combined. Carefully fold in the blueberries.
6. Spoon batter evenly into each muffin paper baking case in muffin tin.
7. Place in the oven for around 20-25mins. Insert a skewer to check they are cooked. Skewer should come out clean.

Prep Time: 10 Minutes

Cook Time: 25 Minutes

Servings: 4

Ingredients

- 1 small mixing bowl
- 1 large bowl
- 1 waffle maker
- 1 organic egg (or 1 chia egg – 1 Tbsp milled chia seeds in 3 Tbsp of water)
- 650 g mash leftover
- 25 g melted (dairy-free) butter
- 3 spring onions
- 1/2 tsp garlic powder

Toppings:

- Raw vegetables (watercress, tomatoes, radishes, avocado, microgreens, cucumber, red onion etc...)
- vegan bacon + maple syrup
- dairy yoghurt + chopped coriander

Instructions

1. Beat the egg in a small bowl (if you are using a chia egg instead, mix the milled chia seeds in 3 Tbsp of water. Set the chia egg aside for 10 mins).
2. Heat your waffle iron to medium-high. I use a setting of 4 on my waffle maker. It has a maximum setting of 7.
3. Place the leftover mash in a large bowl. Add melted (dairy-free) butter, finely chopped spring onions and garlic powder. Mix all together with either the beaten egg or the chia egg. If you feel the mixture is a bit too dry (this can happen if your leftover mash is a few days old) add a splash of plant-based milk.
4. When your waffle iron is hot enough, and you are ready to cook your first waffle, make sure you grease the waffle plates really well.
5. Spread some of the mash mixture in order to cover 3/4 of the waffle plate. Close and cook for 5 minutes until crisp and golden. Conveniently, my waffle maker beeps to let me know the waffles are ready! Do not open the waffle iron while the waffle is cooking.
6. When done transfer the waffle to a rack and keep warm while you are making the rest of the waffles.
7. Serve warm, topped with your favourite ingredients.

8. Pictures above include a waffle loaded with watercress, tomatoes, avocado, vegan bacon and maple syrup and another waffle loaded with watercress, herby dairy-free yoghurt, tomatoes, cucumber, radish, red onion, avocado and microgreens.

Prep Time: 10 Minutes

Cook Time: 25 Minutes

Servings: 4

Ingredients

- 1 mixing bowl
- 1 non-stick pan
- 1 Frying pan
- For The Flatbreads:
- 250 g plain flour
- 2 tsp baking powder
- 1/2 tsp salt
- 200 g dairy-free yoghurt
- 2 tsp vegetable oil

Toppings:

- Vegetable oil
- 8 organic eggs
- 8 tbsp kimchi
- 100 g cheddar, grated
- dill

- yoghurt (optional)

Instructions

1. In a bowl mix together the flour, baking powder, and salt. Add the yoghurt and oil and knead until you have a smooth and elastic dough. Add a bit more flour if the dough is too wet or a bit more yoghurt if the dough is too dry. Cover and set aside for 20 mins to rest.
2. Cut the dough into 4 even balls. Add flour to your working surface and roll out each dough ball to an oval shape of around 3-4mm thickness (1/8 inch).
3. Heat a non-stick pan on high. When the pan is very hot, place the first flatbread in it. Do not use any oil or grease, simply cook the flatbread for 2 mins or so on each side until it starts to char. When done, keep it covered in a warm oven while you cook the rest of the flatbreads.
4. Put some oil in a large frying pan. Working two eggs at a time, start frying the eggs.
5. Put the grill on high. Spread 2 tablespoons of kimchi on each flatbread. Top with some grated cheese. Place each flatbread under the grill for 30 seconds to 1 minute until the cheese starts to melt.

6. Remove from the grill, and place 2 fried eggs on top of each flatbread. Top with dill and (if using) yogurt. Eat straight away.

Prep Time: 10 Minutes

Cook Time: 25 Minutes

Servings: 6

Ingredients

- 2 mixing bowls
- whisk
- pancake pan
- 250 g ricotta
- 300 ml almond milk
- 2 organic eggs – yolk and white separated
- 2 Tbsp melted coconut oil
- 3 Tbsp maple syrup
- 1 tsp vanilla extract
- 250 g wholemeal spelt flour (or use 1/2 wholemeal spelt flour 1/2 white flour or use only white flour)
- 1 tsp baking powder
- 1/2 tsp baking soda
- 1/4 tsp salt

To Serve:

- fresh strawberries
- yoghurt
- almonds
- cocoa nibs
- butter to cook the pancakes

Instructions

1. In a large bowl, mix together ricotta, milk, egg yolks, coconut oil, maple syrup and vanilla.
2. In a separate bowl, mix together spelt flour, salt, baking soda and baking powder.
3. Add the flour mixture into the ricotta mix, blending gently until smooth.
4. Whisk egg white until stiff. Fold into the pancake batter.
5. Cook 2 to 3 pancakes at a time (each should be about 3/4 of a small ladle or 2-3 Tbsp of batter) in a hot pancake pan greased with butter. Do not spread the batter too thin, so you have thick and fluffy pancakes.
6. Cook each pancake for around 2 minutes on one side until the edges look firm and the batter in the middle is a little bubbly. Then flip each pancake on the other

side and cook until golden. Grease the pan between each batch of pancakes.

7. Keep cooked pancakes warm in the oven while you are making the others.

8. Serve these pancakes with fresh strawberry, yoghurt, almonds and cocoa nibs on top.

11. Cauliflower Steak with Salsa Verde

Prep Time: 10 Minutes

Cook Time: 15 Minutes

Servings: 2

Ingredients

- 1 oven tray
- 3 mixing bowls
- 1 medium cauliflower
- Olive oil
- Salsa Verde:
- 30 g basil
- 30 g parsley
- 10 g mint leaves
- 30 g capers
- 1 tsp Dijon mustard
- 75 ml olive oil
- Juice of 1/2 lemon
- 1 garlic clove

White Bean Salad:

- 400 g can of cannellini beans
- 6 cherry tomatoes
- 1/4 small red onion
- 1 Tbsp finely chopped parsley
- 1 garlic clove minced
- 1 Tbsp olive oil
- 1 Tbsp lemon juice
- Salt & pepper

Instructions

1. Preheat the oven to 220°C / fan oven 200°C / 425°F / gas 7.
2. Slice the cauliflower in half from the middle. Cut each half into 2.5cm [1 inch] thick slices. The slices cut from the middle will hold together thanks to the stem of the cauliflower. Do not worry if some of the slices cut from the outer parts of the cauliflower head fall apart. You can roast these florets anyway.
3. Brush the cauliflower steaks (and florets) with some olive oil and place them on an oven tray. Roast for 15 mins on each side until the cauliflower steaks are tender and golden.

4. In the meantime, prepare the salsa verde and white bean salad.

5. For the salsa verde, chop the herbs finely. Place in a mixing bowl with the finely chopped capers, Dijon mustard, olive oil, lemon juice and grated garlic clove. Set aside.

6. Rinse and drain the white beans and place them in a bowl. Add the tomatoes cut in quarters, finely chopped red onion, finely chopped parsley and grated garlic clove. Toss the salad in olive oil and lemon juice. Season to taste with salt and pepper.

7. Place the cooked cauliflower steaks on serving plates. Add some salsa verde on top and some white bean salad on the side. Eat straight away.

Prep Time: 10 Minutes

Cook Time: 45 Minutes

Servings: 12

Ingredients

- tofu press (optional)
- large frying pan
- 12-hole non-stick muffin tin
- Blender
- 390 g extra firm tofu
- 1 onion
- 4 garlic cloves
- 100 g leek
- 260 g baby spinach
- 4 Tbsp chopped parsley
- 2 Tbsp chopped mint
- 2 Tbsp chopped dill
- 100 g sundried tomatoes in oil
- 100 g walnuts
- 4 Tbsp mushroom ketchup
- nutmeg

- lemon juice

- pepper

- 500 g vegan puff pastry

- dairy-free milk

Instructions

1. Press the tofu for around 15 minutes to extract as much water as possible. You can use a tofu press or wrap the tofu in a clean towel and press it between 2 plates by securely placing something heavy on top.
2. Cut the leek in half lengthwise, then cut each half into very thin slices. Set aside
3. Heat 2 Tbsp of the sundried tomatoes oil in a large frying pan.
4. Add finely chopped onion and grated garlic. Fry gently until soft.
5. Add the thinly sliced leeks and cook covered for around 10 minutes until soft.
6. Add roughly chopped spinach to the frying pan and cook until wilted.
7. Preheat the oven to 200C/fan 180C/gas 6.
8. Crumbled the pressed tofu with a fork. When the spinach is wilted, add the crumbled tofu to the pan,

along with the thinly chopped parsley, dill, mint and sundried tomatoes.

9. Grind the walnuts in a blender and add to the vegetable mixture.

10. Add mushroom ketchup. Season to taste with nutmeg, lemon juice and pepper. Remove from heat and set aside.

11. Roll out the puff pastry to a large 36x48cm [14.2 x 19 inches] rectangle. Cut it in twelve squares of 12x12cm [4.75 x 4.75 inches].

12. Grease the hole and top of a non-stick muffin tin with oil.

13. Carefully place the puff pastry squares into the muffin tin holes. Spoon the vegetable and tofu mixture to fill each puff pastry casing evenly.

14. Scrunch up any extra puff pastry towards the inside of each quiche. (if you leave too much pastry hanging outside, you might have issues removing the cooked quiches from the muffin tin).

15. Brush some dairy-free milk on top of the pastry.

16. Bake in the oven for 20 to 25 minutes until the pastry is golden. When done, remove from the oven and let the quiches stand for 10 minutes on the muffin tin.

17. Carefully remove each quiche from the muffin tin and place on a serving dish.

18. Serve hot or cold. If desired, add some extra walnuts and herbs on top before serving.

Prep Time: 10 Minutes

Cook Time: 45 Minutes

Servings: 6

Ingredients

- Large shallow casserole
- 4 tbsp olive oil
- 1 medium onion
- 2 garlic cloves
- 1 Tbsp ginger grated
- 2 tsp ground coriander
- 500 g green cabbage head
- 275 g tomatoes
- 2 stalks of lemongrass
- 2 kaffir leaves
- 250 ml vegetable stock
- 1 Tbsp tomato paste
- 150 g jasmine rice (10 minutes cook)
- 400 ml light coconut milk
- 250 ml vegetable stock
- 1 Tbsp tamari sauce

- 400 g can aduki beans
- 30 g fresh coriander
- lime juice

To Serve:

- 2 limes
- 1 red chilli

Instructions

1. Chop the cabbage finely. Cut each tomato into 8 cubes. Bash the lemongrass to bruise the stalks.
2. Heat some olive oil in a large casserole.
3. Add finely chopped onion and fry gently until soft. Add crushed garlic cloves, grated ginger and ground coriander. Fry for another couple of minutes.
4. Add the finely chopped cabbage, cubed tomatoes, bruised lemongrass, kaffir leaves and 250ml (US 1cup) of vegetable stock. Bring to the boil, then cook covered under medium heat for 30 minutes until the cabbage is cooked. Stir from time to time so that the cabbage does not stick to the bottom of the pan.
5. Add the tomato paste, rice, coconut milk, 250ml (US 1cup) of vegetable stock and 1 Tbsp of tamari. Mix

well all together. Bring to the boil, then cook covered under medium heat for 15 minutes. Stir from time to time so that the cabbage and rice do not stick to the bottom of the pan.

6. Wash and drain the aduki beans. Mix them into the cabbage and rice mixture along with the finely chopped coriander. Season with lime juice, a bit more tamari sauce if needed and some salt.

7. Remove the lemongrass stalks. Serve with some extra lime juice and chopped fresh red chillies on top.

Prep Time: 10 Minutes

Cook Time: 40 Minutes

Servings: 4

Ingredients

- roasting tray
- Blender
- mixing bowl
- 750 g new potatoes
- 4 Tbsp olive oil
- Juice of 1 lemon
- 2 Tbsp chopped rosemary
- 250 g on-the-vine cherry tomatoes
- 4 garlic cloves slivered

Butter Bean Dip:

- 400 g can butter beans
- 2 Tbsp tahini
- 2 garlic cloves
- 1 tsp ground cumin

- 4 Tbsp water

- 3 Tbsp lemon juice to taste

- ½ to 1 tsp salt

- 2 Tbsp extra-virgin olive oil

Instructions

1. Heat some water in a large pan. When boiling add the potatoes and part-boil them for 10 mins. When done, drain and set aside to cool.

2. Preheat the oven to 220C/fan 200C/gas 7.

3. Depending on their size, cut the potatoes in halves or quarters.

4. In a bowl, mix together the olive oil, the juice of one lemon and the chopped rosemary.

5. Spread the potatoes on a baking tray and toss in the oil and rosemary mixture.

6. Cook for 15 mins then add the tomatoes and slivered garlic cloves, tossing everything into the oil and rosemary mixture. Return the baking tray to the oven and cook for a further 20 mins. Keep an eye from time to time as cooking will depend on the size of the potatoes. If the tomatoes cook faster, take them out of

the oven and set them aside until the potatoes are cooked.

7. Make the dip while the vegetables are in the oven. Place drained and rinsed butter beans in a blender. Add tahini, garlic cloves, cumin and water. Whizz to a paste. Add lemon juice and salt to taste. Whizz again with some olive oil. You can adjust the amount of water to get your desired consistency.

8. Once the vegetables are cooked, spread the butter bean dip on a serving dish. Drizzle some extra olive oil on top. Top with the roasted potatoes and tomatoes. Season the vegetables to taste with salt and pepper.

9. Serve warm or at room temperature.

Prep Time: 15 Minutes

Cook Time: 25 Minutes

Servings: 4

Ingredients

- 400 g baby aubergines
- vegetable oil and/or coconut oil
- 1 onion finely chopped
- 3 garlic cloves grated
- 1 red pepper - deseeded and diced
- 1 Tbsp grated fresh ginger
- 1 Tbsp garam masala + 1/2 tsp
- 1 tsp ground cinnamon
- 1/2 tsp chilli flakes
- 1 tsp turmeric
- 1 Tbsp tomato puree
- 3 curry leaves
- 400 g can chopped tomatoes
- one handful of raisins
- 400 ml coconut milk
- 400 g can chickpeas

- lemon juice to taste

- salt & pepper

- 1-2 tsp sugar optional

To Serve:

- Rice

- Loaf bread

- bunch of fresh coriander

- fresh chilli

Instructions

1. Preheat the oven to 200°C / 180°C Fan / Gas 6.
2. Cut the baby aubergines in half lengthwise. Spread them on a roasting tray. Drizzle with some vegetable oil. Cook for 20-25mins until soft. Set aside when done
3. In the meantime, heat some vegetable oil (or coconut oil) in a large saucepan. Add the finely chopped onion and grated garlic. Fry gently until soft.
4. Add the diced red pepper, grated ginger, garam masala, ground cinnamon, ground turmeric, chilli flakes, tomato puree and curry leaves. Gently fry together for 3 minutes. Add chopped tomatoes, raisins

and coconut milk. Simmer for 10-15mins until the sauce has thickened.

5. Add the chickpeas and the baby aubergines to the pan. Season to taste with lemon juice plus salt and pepper. Add 1/2 tsp garam masala (optional). Carry on simmering the curry for 10 minutes or so. If you find the curry too acidic, add some sugar as needed.

6. Serve with rice, naan bread, fresh chilli and plenty of freshly chopped coriander.

16. Cabbage & Carrot Fritters

Prep Time: 20 Minutes

Cook Time: 15 Minutes

Servings: 8

Ingredients

- salad bowl
- Frying pan
- 150 g green cabbage – finely chopped
- 175 g carrots – grated on the coarse side of a cheese grater
- 2 organic eggs beaten
- 100 g plain flour
- 2 Tbsp freshly grated ginger
- 2 Tbsp chopped mint
- 2 Tbsp chopped coriander
- 1 tsp garlic powder
- 1 Tbsp soy sauce
- juice of 1 lime
- 1 tsp ground cumin
- 1/2 tsp salt
- vegetable oil to fry

Dipping Sauce:

- 2 Tbsp sweet chilli sauce
- 2 Tbsp rice vinegar
- 2 Tbsp toasted sesame oil
- 2 Tbsp lime juice
- 1 tsp tamari sauce
- 2 tsp dark brown sugar
- 1 Tbsp freshly chopped mint

To Serve:

- spring onions
- red chilli
- dairy-free yoghurt

Instructions

1. In a large salad bowl mix together the finely chopped cabbage, grated carrot, beaten eggs, flour, grated ginger, chopped mint, chopped coriander, garlic powder, soy sauce, lime juice, ground cumin and salt. Once the mixture is well blended set aside for 10 mins.
2. Prepare the dipping sauce by mixing together in a bowl the sweet chilli sauce, rice vinegar, toasted

sesame oil, lime juice, tamari sauce, dark brown sugar and freshly chopped mint.

3. Get a large, deep frying pan and fill it with vegetable oil (you need the oil level to be around 2cm [0.8 inches] high). When the oil is hot, spoon 1 generous tablespoon of vegetable mixture in the pan (to make sure the fritters are evenly shaped I use a round cookie cutter as a guide, adding the vegetable mixture inside the cookie-cutter). Flatten the top of the fritter. Repeat to make a second fritter. Depending on the size of your pan, you should be able to cook 3 to 4 fritters at once.

4. Cook for 2 to 3 mins until you can flip the fritters on the other side. When the fritters are golden, transfer to a side plate lined with some paper towel until you cook the rest.

5. Serve the fritters warm topped with chopped spring onion, red chilli peppers and (dairy-free) yoghurt as well as the dipping sauce on the side.

Prep Time: 10 Minutes

Cook Time: 15 Minutes

Servings: 4

Ingredients

- saucepan
- 2 Tbsp vegetable oil or coconut oil
- 1 large onion
- 3 garlic cloves
- 1 Tbsp grated ginger
- 300 g tomatoes – roughly chopped in small dice
- 1 1/2 Tbsp garam masala
- 1 tsp turmeric
- 1 tsp chilli powder
- 250 ml vegetable stock
- 400 ml can coconut milk
- 450 g broccoli florets
- 400 g can chickpeas
- 3 Tbsp crunchy peanut butter
- lemon juice to taste
- salt

To Serve:

- peanuts
- fresh coriander
- red chillies
- rice

Instructions

1. Heat the oil in a large saucepan. Add finely chopped onion and crushed garlic. Fry gently until soft.
2. Add grated ginger, chopped tomatoes and fry gently together for a couple of minutes.
3. Add garam masala, turmeric, chilli powder, vegetable stock and coconut milk to the pan. Stir until everything is well blended. Add the broccoli florets cut in medium size. Bring the boil, then stirring the broccoli from time to time, cook covered under medium heat for 10-12 minutes. The broccoli should be cooked but still have a bite.
4. Add the peanut butter to the saucepan making sure that it melts in the curry sauce so there are no lumps. Add the chickpeas and cook for another minute or so.
5. Season to taste with lemon juice and salt.

6. Serve this broccoli curry with rice, topped with crushed peanuts, fresh coriander and sliced red chillies.

Prep Time: 20 Minutes

Cook Time: 30 Minutes

Servings: 4

Ingredients

For The Flatbreads:

- 300 g plain flour
- 2 tsp baking powder
- 1 tsp salt
- 1 Tbsp olive oil
- 300 g dairy-free yoghurt or plain dairy yoghurt
- For The Roasted Cauliflower:
- 1 small cauliflower – approx 600g / 1.3 lbs
- olive oil
- Salt

To Serve:

- rocket leaves
- dairy-free yoghurt or plain dairy yoghurt
- chilli flakes
- Lemon juice

Instructions

1. In a bowl mix together the flour, baking powder and salt. Add the yoghurt and olive oil and knead until you have a smooth and elastic dough. Add a bit more flour if the dough is too wet. Cover and set aside for 20 mins to rest.

2. Preheat the oven to 200°C / 180°C Fan / Gas 6.

3. Make the muhammara dip by following this recipe. Set aside when done.

4. Cut the cauliflower into medium chunk florets. Spread on a baking tray. Drizzle some olive oil on top and add a little bit of salt. Place the tray in the oven and roast the cauliflower for 25-30 mins until golden. Keep warm when done.

5. While the cauliflower is in the oven, you can start cooking the flatbreads. Cut the dough into 6 even balls. Add flour to your working surface and roll out each dough ball to a 21-23cm circle [8-9"].

6. Heat a non-stick pan on high. When the pan is very hot, place the first flatbread in it. Do not use any oil or grease, simply cook the flatbread 2 mins or so on each side until it starts to char. When done, keep it covered in a warm oven while you cook the rest of the flatbreads.

7. When ready to serve, spread some muhammara dip on each flatbread. Add some roasted cauliflower on top. Top with some rocket leaves, yoghurt, chilli flakes and extra lemon juice.

Prep Time: 10 Minutes

Cook Time: 30 Minutes

Servings: 2

Ingredients

- 1 large frying pan
- 4 Tbsp olive oil
- 1 medium red onion
- 250 g courgettes
- 250 g tomatoes (cherry or baby plums)
- 2 garlic cloves crushed
- 1 1/2 tsp dry mixed Italian herbs
- 400 g vegan potato gnocchi
- 1 generous handful of black olives
- 90 g roasted red pepper from a jar
- salt & pepper
- 1 small bunch of basil
- Optional
- vegan parmesan
- or vegetarian parmesan

Instructions

1. Cut the red onion into thin slices. Cut the courgettes into thin slices and cut each slice into quarters. Cut the tomatoes in halves.
2. Heat 2 Tbsp of olive oil in a large frying pan. Gently fry the red onion slices until soft (around 5 mins).
3. Add the sliced courgettes, tomatoes, crushed garlic cloves and dry mixed Italian herbs. Fry under medium heat for 10-15mins until the vegetables are cooked.
4. Once done, transfer vegetable mixture to a plate.
5. Add 2 Tbsp of olive oil to the frying pan. Add the gnocchi and fry under medium heat until golden and crunchy.
6. Return the vegetables to the pan with the gnocchi and reheat altogether.
7. Add the olives cut in halves and the roasted red pepper cut into thin slices.
8. Season to taste with salt and pepper. Serve straightaway with some fresh basil on top. If desired you can also add a sprinkle of vegan or vegetarian parmesan.

Prep Time: 10 Minutes

Cook Time: 25 Minutes

Servings: 4

Ingredients

- large saucepan
- 2 Tbsp vegetable oil (or melted coconut oil)
- 1 onion
- 5 garlic
- 3 cm fresh ginger root
- 2 tsp ground coriander
- 2 tsp ground cumin
- 1 tsp ground cinnamon
- 1 tsp chilli powder
- 1 tsp turmeric
- 150 g baby plum tomatoes
- 800 g can chickpeas
- 400 g can chopped tomatoes
- 400 ml can coconut milk
- 125 g bunch of kale or spinach (hard stem removed)
- 1/2 tsp garam masala

- lemon juice to taste
- salt

To Serve:

- fresh coriander
- dairy-free yoghurt
- chilli flakes

Instructions

1. Heat the oil in a large saucepan. Add the finely chopped onion and fry gently until soft.
2. Add the minced garlic cloves, grated ginger root, coriander, cumin, cinnamon, chilli powder and turmeric.
3. Add the tomatoes cut in halves. Fry gently altogether until the tomatoes are soft.
4. Add the chickpeas, chopped tomatoes and coconut milk. Bring to the boil and cook covered under medium heat for 10 minutes.
5. Add the kale (roughly chopped) and carry on cooking covered under medium heat for another 8 to 10 minutes until kale is cooked.

6. When done, add ½ tsp garam masala. Season to taste with lemon juice and salt.

7. Serve with rice, topped with fresh coriander, dairy-free yoghurt and chilli flakes.

21. Flatbreads with Harissa Mushrooms

Prep Time: 10 Minutes

Cook Time: 30 Minutes

Servings: 4

Ingredients

- 2 large frying pans
- 1 mixing bowl
- 1 Rolling Pin
- For The Flatbreads:
- 350 g self-raising flour
- 1 tsp salt
- 300 g dairy-free yoghurt
- 1 Tbsp olive oil

For The Harissa Mushrooms:

- 2 Tbsp olive oil
- 80 g red onion
- 2 garlic cloves
- 1 red pepper, diced

- 250 g mushrooms, sliced
- 400 g can chopped tomatoes
- 1 tsp cumin
- 1 tsp smoked paprika
- 3 Tbsp rose harissa
- 400 g can chickpeas
- 1 small handful of chopped coriander leaves
- lemon juice to taste
- Salt

To Serve:

- dairy-free yoghurt
- fresh coriander

Instructions

1. In a bowl mix together the flour and salt. Add the yoghurt and olive oil and knead until you have a smooth and elastic dough. Add a bit more flour if the dough is too wet or a bit more yoghurt if the dough is too dry. Cover and set aside for 20 mins to rest.
2. You can start making the harissa mushrooms while the flatbread dough is resting.

3. Heat some olive in a large frying pan. Add the finely chopped onion and the crushed garlic. Fry gently until soft.

4. Add the diced pepper and the sliced mushrooms. Fry on medium to high heat until the mushrooms start to soften.

5. Add the chopped tomatoes, drained chickpeas, cumin, smoked paprika and rose harissa. Simmer on medium heat until the mushrooms and pepper are cooked and the sauce has thickened. Reduce the heat to low if you feel the vegetables are becoming too dry.

6. While the mushrooms are cooking, you can start cooking the flatbreads.

7. Cut the dough into 4 even balls. Add flour to your working surface and roll out each dough ball to a 20cm / 8 inches circle.

8. Heat a non-stick pan on high. When the pan is very hot, place the first flatbread in it. Do not use any oil or grease, simply cook the flatbread 2 mins or so on each side until it starts to char. When done, keep it covered in a warm oven while you cook the rest of the flatbreads.

9. Just before serving, add a handful of chopped coriander leaves to the harissa mushrooms. Season to taste with lemon juice and salt.

10. Place some harissa mushrooms on top of each flatbread. Top with some yoghurt and fresh coriander.

Prep Time: 10 Minutes

Cook Time: 30 Minutes

Servings: 4

Ingredients

- 1 large saucepan
- 2 Tbsp olive oil
- 1 large onion
- 1 yellow pepper
- 1 red chilli
- 1 tsp smoked paprika
- 2 tsp ground cumin
- 2 tsp ground coriander
- 500 g Quorn Mince
- 400 g can chopped tomatoes
- 3 Tbsp tomato purée
- 750 ml vegetable stock
- 3 garlic cloves
- 1 tsp dried oregano
- 400 g can kidney beans
- 2 tsp cornflour

- 1 tsp sugar

- lime or lemon juice to taste

- salt to taste

To Serve:

- fresh coriander

- guacamole

- (dairy-free) yoghurt or soured cream

- tortilla chips

- extra chilli

Instructions

1. Heat the olive oil in a large saucepan.
2. Add the finely chopped onion and fry gently until soft.
3. Deseed the yellow pepper and cut it in 1cm [0.4 inches] dice.
4. Add the smoked paprika, ground cumin, ground coriander, diced pepper and finely chopped chilli to the pan. Fry gently for a minute or so.
5. Add the Quorn mince, chopped tomatoes, tomato purée, stock, grated garlic and oregano to the pan. Stir well. Bring to the boil, then cook uncovered under medium heat for 15 mins.

6. Rinse and drain the kidney beans.

7. Put 3 tablespoons of the chilli sauce in a small glass and mix in 2 teaspoons of cornflour. Return the mixture to the pan.

8. Add the kidney beans into the chilli. Cook under medium heat for another 5 minutes or so, until the chilli sauce has thickened.

9. Season to taste with sugar, lemon or lime juice and salt.

10. Serve with rice topped with tortilla chips, fresh coriander, guacamole, (dairy-free) yoghurt or sour cream, and some extra chilli.

Prep Time: 10 Minutes

Cook Time: 30 Minutes

Servings: 4

Ingredients

- roasting tray
- 800 g sweet potatoes
- 3 Tbsp olive oil
- ½ tsp smoked paprika
- ½ tsp salt
- 8-12 mini tortilla wraps

Toppings:

- Charred Corn Salsa
- Avocado Mayo
- freshly chopped coriander
- lime juice
- red chilli

Instructions

1. Preheat oven to 220C/200C fan/gas 7.
2. Peel sweet potatoes and cut them into 1cm [0.4 inches] thick slices. Place in a bowl with olive oil, smoked paprika and salt. Toss well until the sweet potatoes are coated all over. Spread on a baking tray and cook for 25mins until soft.
3. While the sweet potatoes are roasting in the oven, prepare the avocado mayo and charred corn salad
4. Once everything is ready, top the tortillas with some roasted sweet potatoes, charred corn salad and avocado mayo.
5. If using, serve with some freshly chopped coriander, lime juice and sliced red chilli.

Prep Time: 15 Minutes

Cook Time: 30 Minutes

Servings: 2

Ingredients

- 1 large frying pan
- 1 Blender
- 1 saucepan

For The Sauce:

- 225 g cauliflower floret
- 2 Tbsp olive oil
- 1/2 small onion
- 2 garlic cloves
- 100 g cooked beetroot
- 1 Tbsp lemon juice
- ½ tsp dried Italian herbs
- 100 ml dairy-free milk
- 2 Tbsp capucine capers
- salt & pepper

Toppings:

- olive oil
- ½ onion
- 1 garlic clove
- 150 g mushrooms
- 100 g spinach leaves
- few capers or caperberries
- lemon juice
- handful of Kalamata olives
- handful of walnuts
- For The Pasta:
- 160 g dry spaghetti

Instructions

1. Heat some salted water in a large saucepan. When boiling, add cauliflower florets and cook for 10 mins until soft and tender. Drain and set aside to cool.
2. While the cauliflower florets are cooking, heat some olive oil in a frying pan. Add half of a finely chopped onion. Fry gently until soft. Add 2 crushed garlic cloves and cook for a few more minutes, taking care not to let the garlic go brown. Set aside in a bowl.
3. Heat some more olive oil in the same frying pan. Add the other half of the onion. Fry gently until soft. Add 1

crushed garlic clove and the finely chopped mushrooms. Fry under medium heat until the mushrooms are soft. Add finely chopped spinach leaves to the pan and cook until wilted. Set aside when done.

4. In the meantime cook the pasta according to packet instructions in a separate saucepan.

5. When the cauliflower has cooled down, place the florets in a blender with the reserved onion and garlic, beetroot, lemon juice, dried Italian herbs, dairy-free milk and capers. Blend to a smooth creamy texture. Season to taste with salt and pepper.

6. Mix cooked pasta and the cauliflower sauce. Share evenly between 2 plates.

7. Serve straight away, topped with the mushrooms and spinach mixture. Add a squeeze of lemon juice, capers or caperberries, Kalamata olives and walnuts on top.

Prep Time: 10 Minutes

Cook Time: 50 Minutes

Servings: 4

Ingredients

- baking tray
- saucepan
- 4 medium sweet potatoes
- olive oil
- 1 onion finely chopped
- 5 garlic cloves grated
- 2 tsp smoked paprika
- 1 tsp ground cumin
- 1 red pepper diced
- 400 g can chopped tomatoes
- 200 g beluga lentils
- 400 ml vegetable stock
- 175 g spinach leaves
- lemon juice to taste

To Serve:

- small bunch fresh coriander
- dairy-free cream or yoghurt

Instructions

1. Heat oven to 200C/180C fan/gas 6.
2. Wash and scrub the sweet potatoes. Place on a baking tray. Pierce all over with a fork. Drizzle some olive on top. Cook for 40-50mins until soft. The cooking time will depend on the size of the sweet potatoes.
3. Heat some olive oil in a saucepan. Add finely chopped onion, grated garlic cloves, smoked paprika and ground cumin. Fry gently until the onion is soft. Add diced red pepper and gently fry for another 2 ins or so. Add lentils, tomatoes and vegetable stock.
4. Bring to boil. Then cook covered under medium heat for 15mins then uncovered for another 15mins.
5. Mix in the spinach leaves and cook for a couple of minutes until wilted. Season to taste with lemon juice, salt and pepper.
6. When the sweet potatoes are cooked, cut them lengthwise down the centre. Spread the sides slightly and top with lentil mix. Serve with plenty of chopped

fresh coriander and a dollop of dairy- free cream or yoghurt.

Prep Time: 10 Minutes

Cook Time: 30 Minutes

Servings: 4

Ingredients

- oven tray
- Blender
- Frying pan
- 500 g butternut squash
- olive oil
- 1 small red onion thinly sliced
- 1 garlic clove
- 200 g spinach

For The Hummus:

- 400 g can chickpeas
- 2 Tbsp tahini
- 3-5 Tbsp water or chickpea brine
- 2 Tbsp olive oil
- 2 garlic cloves
- 1 tsp ground cumin

- 1/2 Tbsp freshly grated ginger
- 2 Tbsp lemon juice

To Serve:

- 4 slices of bread
- harissa

Instructions

1. Preheat the oven to 200C/fan 180C/gas 6.
2. Peel the butternut and cut in small dice. Spread the butternut dice on an oven tray. Drizzle with some olive oil. Cook for 30-35mins until soft and golden.
3. In the meantime, make the hummus by whizzing together drained chickpeas, tahini, garlic, lemon juice, ginger, olive oil, and ground cumin. Add water or chickpea brine to get your desire consistency. Season to taste with salt.
4. Heat some olive oil in a large frying pan. Add finely chopped red onion and crushed garlic clove. Fry gently until soft. Add spinach and cook until wilted. Season to taste with salt. Set aside.
5. When the butternut is ready, toast the bread slices.

6. Add a generous amount of hummus on each slice of bread. Top with the spinach mixture. Share the butternut evenly between each portion. Serve warm with a drizzle of harissa on top.

Prep Time: 10 Minutes

Cook Time: 30 Minutes

Servings: 4

Ingredients

- baking tray
- bowl
- 600 g parsnips
- olive oil
- 3 fresh sprigs of thyme
- 75 g pecan nuts
- 1 orange either blood orange or regular orange

For The Tahini Dressing:

- 1 Tbsp tahini
- 5 Tbsp dairy-free yoghurt
- 1 garlic clove grated
- 1 tsp ground cumin
- 1/2 tsp ground cinnamon
- 2-3 Tbsp lemon juice
- 3 Tbsp water

- 1 Tbsp maple syrup or agave syrup or honey if vegetarian

To Serve:

- handful of freshly chopped parsley

Instructions

1. Preheat oven to 200C/fan 180C/gas 6.
2. Peel parsnips and cut into long sticks. Spread the parsnip sticks and thyme sprigs on a baking tray. Drizzle with some olive oil. Cook for 20mins, then add the pecan nuts to the tray and carry on cooking for another 8-10mins until parsnip is golden.
3. In the meantime make the tahini dressing by mixing together tahini, yoghurt, garlic, ground cumin, cinnamon, lemon juice, water, maple syrup, salt and pepper. Adjust seasoning and thickness to suit your own taste.
4. Peel the orange. Slice and cut into small chunks.
5. Once the parnsips are cooked, toss in the orange chunks and freshly chopped parsley.
6. Serve the salad straight away so it can be eaten warm with a generous drizzle of tahini dressing on top.

Prep Time: 10 Minutes

Cook Time: 35 Minutes

Servings: 4

Ingredients

- Frying pan
- saucepan
- 750 g baby potatoes
- olive oil
- 1 onion
- 2 garlic cloves
- 1 red pepper
- 2 tsp dried thyme
- 2 x180g packs of Like Meat "Like Smoked Sausage" [2 x 6.3 oz]
- 2 handfuls baby spinach leaves
- lemon juice
- salt & pepper
- small bunch of parsley

Instructions

1. Cut the baby potatoes in halves. Cut the sausages into slices.

2. Heat some water in a large pan. When the water is boiling, transfer the potatoes to the pan and cook for around 10-12mins until cooked. Drain well when done.

3. Heat some olive oil in a large frying pan. Fry the boiled potatoes until golden all over. You might have to do this by batches. When the potatoes are done, transfer them to a plate.

4. Heat some more olive oil in the frying pan. Add finely chopped onion, crushed garlic cloves, sliced red pepper and thyme. Cook for 3 mins or so until the onion is soft. Add the sliced sausages and cook together for 6-8 mins.

5. Add the fried potatoes back into the pan, followed by the spinach. Stir all together and cook until the spinach is wilted and the potatoes have warmed up. Season to taste with lemon juice, salt & pepper. Serve straight away with some freshly chopped parsley on top.

Prep Time: 10 Minutes

Cook Time: 35 Minutes

Servings: 6

Ingredients

- baking tray
- large saucepan
- olive oil
- 1 onion
- 4 garlic cloves
- 2 tsp ground coriander
- 2 tsp ground cumin
- 1 tsp ground turmeric
- 1 Tbsp freshly grated ginger
- 1/2 tsp smoked paprika
- 1 tsp ground cinnamon
- 1 tsp chilli powder
- 500 g sweet potato
- 1 small red pepper
- 400 g can chopped tomatoes
- 750 ml vegetable stock

- lemon juice

Toppings:

- 400 g can chickpeas
- olive oil
- fresh coriander
- harissa paste
- dairy-free yoghurt or cream

Instructions

For The Crunchy Chickpeas:

1. Heat oven to 180C/160C fan/gas 4. Toss the drained chickpeas in some olive oil and 1/2 tsp of salt. Spread on a baking tray. Cook for around 30-35mins until crunchy

For The Soup

1. Heat some olive oil in a large saucepan. Add finely chopped onion and crushed garlic. Fry gently until soft.

2. Add ground coriander, cumin, turmeric, freshly grated ginger, smoked paprika, ground cinnamon and

chilli powder. Fry gently for another couple of minutes.

3. Add peeled sweet potatoes cut into small dice and red pepper roughly chopped. Add chopped tomatoes and vegetable stock. Bring to the boil. Reduce heat to medium and cook covered for around 20mins until sweet potatoes are cooked.

4. Liquidise the soup until smooth. Season with lemon juice and salt.

5. Serve this soup topped with crunchy chickpeas, harissa, chopped fresh coriander and some dairy-free yoghurt or cream.

Prep Time: 10 Minutes

Cook Time: 35 Minutes

Servings: 4

Ingredients

- 2 medium aubergines
- 2 red onion
- 2 red pepper
- 2 green pepper
- 4 vine tomatoes
- 2 shallots
- 4 garlic cloves
- 1 green chilli
- 2 tsp sugar
- 2 Tbsp tomato puree
- 200 g bulgur wheat
- 2 tsp vegetable stock powder
- 20 g bunch of basil
- 20 g bunch of coriander
- 20 g bunch of flat leaf parsley
- 50 g walnuts

- salt & pepper

- olive oil

Instructions

1. Preheat oven to 200C/fan 180C/gas 6. Trim the aubergine then halve lengthways. Chop each half into four long strips then chop widthways into 2cm [0.8 inches] pieces. Pop on a baking tray, drizzle with oil and season with salt and pepper. Toss to coat then spread out in one layer and roast on the top shelf of your oven until soft and golden, 15-20 mins.

2. Halve, peel and finely slice the shallot. and the red onion. Peel and grate the garlic (or use a garlic press). Halve the peppers and discard the cores and seeds. Chop into roughly 2cm [0.8 inches] pieces. Chop the vine tomato into roughly 2cm [0.8 inches] pieces. Halve the chilli lengthways, remove the seeds then finely chop.

3. Heat a drizzle of oil in a large saucepan on medium heat and add the shallot. Cook, stirring, until softened, 2-3 mins, then stir in the tomato purée and bulgur wheat. Add half the stock powder and 250ml of water [8.45 fl oz / US 1 cup] for the bulgur, stir and

bring to the boil. Pop a lid on the pan and remove from the heat. Leave to the side for 12-15 mins or until ready to serve.

4. Meanwhile, heat a drizzle of oil in a large frying pan on medium heat. When hot, add the onion and a pinch of salt and cook, stirring occasionally, until soft , 3-4 mins. Stir in the garlic, peppers and a pinch of chilli (go easy on the chilli – you can add more later!) and cook for another minute.

5. Next, stir in the tomato, 100ml of water [3.4 fl oz], remaining stock powder and sugar. Pop a lid on the pan and lower the heat to medium-low. Leave to simmer until thick and tomatoey with the peppers just soft, 5-6 mins. TIP: The stew should have some texture to it; we don't want mush!

6. Roughly chop the basil, parsley and coriander (stalks and all). Roughly chop the walnuts. Stir the walnuts and half the herbs through the bulgur. Season to taste with salt and pepper if needed. Stir the roasted aubergine and remaining herbs through the stew. Season to taste with salt and pepper. Ajapsandali done! Serve the bulgur in bowls topped with the Ajapsandali – finish with a sprinkling of chilli if liked. Enjoy!